Stop Drinking Alcohol in 5 Steps

Discover Effective Ways to Quit Drinking and Stop Alcohol Abuse

Helen Wright

Copyright © 2019 Helen Wright

All rights reserved.

DEDICATION

To my heroes, who choose to fight for a better life.

Table of Contents

Introduction 1

    What will you discover in this book and how it will help?... 2

    The importance of reading this book and applying new things 2

The Stages of Alcoholism 4

    Stage 1: pre-alcoholic 4

    Stage 2: early alcoholic 4

    Stage 3: middle alcoholic 5

    Stage 4: late alcoholic 5

    Am I an alcoholic? 6

    Signs that you may be an alcoholic 7

At the Bottom of the Bottle 9

    What can happen with an alcoholic? 9

    Effect on health 10

    How does alcohol affect your senses? 11

    Sight 12

    Taste and smell 13

    Touch 13

Hearing 14

Causes of Alcoholism 15

Easy access and availability.. 15

Mass media effect 16

Boredom 17

The Power of Our Beliefs 19

Why do we like to drink?... 19

Myths 20

Awareness of the problem... 21

Reasons to Quit Drinking 24

Feeling better...24

Looking younger 25

Saving money 26

Social stability 26

A healthy heart 27

Gain time for taking up new activities 28

Health improvement 29

Focus on personal achievements and development 30

Why Quitting Can Be So Hard? 31

There is no magic pill 31

Admitting you have a problem 31

Fear of recovery 32

Brain changes 32

Rules to Follow on This Path 35

First rule: change your lifestyle 35

Second rule: be completely honest 36

Third rule: ask for help 36

Fourth rule: practice self-care 37

Fifth rule: do not bend the rules 38

The Ups and Downs of Real People 39

It is never too late 39

Fight for your family 40

There is no shame in seeking help 41

Find your passion 42

Make changes happen in 5 steps 43

Build motivation 43

Avoid temptation 44

Practice self-consciousness 45

Pursue the self-development goal 45

Willpower only does not work 46

Conclusion **48**

Introduction

Are you sick of the effects of drinking on your life? Do you have even a tiny shred of desire to stop drinking? This book is written from the heart and contains brutally honest techniques that can save you from a self-destructive path of alcoholism.

Alcohol addiction is by no means a simple problem, with millions of people around the world struggling with this issue. Approximately 88,000 people end up dying each year from problems related to alcohol in the US. Alcohol is second only to tobacco, as well as sedentary lifestyle or a poor diet being the most avoidable reason of death in the nation. Of all driving fatalities, alcohol-impaired driving is responsible for over 30% of all fatalities as drunk driving costs the US over $199 billion each year. With approximately 15 million people struggling with disorders related to alcohol in the US, it comes with no surprise that only 8% of these people receive treatment.

The Center for Disease Control and Prevention (CDC) report further highlights that approximately 4,700 teens die due to alcohol use every year, which is a figure that eclipses the combined teen fatalities from all illegal drugs. Even more worrying is the fact that over 65 million people in America seem to practice binge drinking within the past month. This figure represents over 40% of the alcohol users currently.

These figures indicate just how wide the problem with alcohol addiction seems to be. Knowledge about every aspect of alcohol addiction is a process tool in combating this problem. This book seeks to equip you with the necessary knowledge to fight off this disaster from your life.

What will you discover in this book and how it will help?

This book draws a clear line between normal drinking and alcoholism. By reading this book, you will be able to understand exactly what you need to do to stop drinking. This is achieved through tackling facts about drinking and exploring sure ways to evade the persistent urge to drink. The impacts of drinking are highlighting in terms of how alcohol consumption affects the brain and the self-help strategies are provided to detach yourself from the tight grasp of addiction. This book investigates empowering you to understand why alcoholics drink the way they do. Many a time, you might be wondering why you or a loved one drinks the way they do and what should be done to stop such reckless and destructive behavior. Well, this book answers those two questions in an easy to understand way.

The importance of reading this book and applying new things

This book will give you clarity on your situation. It will open your eyes to new facts so that you will understand that you hold power to control and change your life. You will also get the skills to deal with social pressure. Alcohol might seem like the center of your social life and entertainment, making it hard to quit. However, the problems that it has brought to your life, relationships, and carrier might be a too high stake. This book helps you to realize the value of leading a responsible and productive life. It opens your eyes to other forms of hobbies and fun activities that do not require drinking. While this book is not a prescription from your general practitioner, reading it will make a significant impact on your life. Applying what you read in your life will not only give you the drive to quit drinking but empower you to make sober decisions to take control of your life daily.

The Stages of Alcoholism

Most people are able to handle moderate consumption of alcohol without any problem. However, certain risk factors can make alcohol consumption an uncontrollable addiction with the alcoholism stages, progressing to a situation where you lose all control unless you undergo proper treatment or intervention. Every alcoholic goes through four defined stages.

Stage 1: pre-alcoholic

Little evidence of alcoholism tendencies can be identified during the pre-alcoholic stage. Typical behaviors to the casual observer characterize this stage with drinking being mainly social. As the stage progresses, a person begins drinking more frequently while also using alcohol as a means for stress reduction. Psychologically, people begin to develop a high tolerance for alcohol, which is characterized by the ability to drink large quantities of alcohol while remaining functional. Inebriation can only develop from larger amounts of alcohol. A critical look at your early behavior including whether you drink to feel better, or when you are only drinking in a social setting when the people around you are also drinking, can help you identify whether you are in a danger of developing an alcohol problem.

Stage 2: early alcoholic

Experiencing your first blackout officially positions you in the early stages of alcoholism. This stage is associated with an increasing discomfort with drinking, which develops alongside the inability to fight the urge for alcohol consumption. Certain behaviors may begin forming during this stage, including lying about drinking and hiding drinks in forms such as spiked coffee or soda. Thought of alcohol can become obsessive as your alcohol tolerance continues to grow. The easiest way to understand if you are already in this stage is by analyzing the social aspect of your drinking to identify if others are noticing some changes in your behavior.

Stage 3: middle alcoholic

The symptoms characterizing an alcoholic will be more obvious at this stage to most family members and friends. You begin missing social obligations and work due to hangovers or drinking episodes. This stage also marks the beginning of drinking at inappropriate times, such as at work or when taking care of children. Strong cravings for alcohol are common in this stage as you also begin withdrawal symptoms such as severe headaches, loss of appetite, rapid heartbeat, enlarged pupils, excessive sweating, tremors, and sharing. Irritable behavior and arguments with friends and family become prominent during this stage. Physical changes can start developing, including facial redness, sluggishness, weight loss or gain, and stomach bloating. Some people try to find help at his stage thresh support groups, which can be an effective strategy of taking control of your life.

Stage 4: late alcoholic

Long-term alcohol abuse culminates into this stage. After-effects of the abuse become more apparent due to the development of serious health problems. Alcohol consumption is adopted as an all-day affair with everything else, taking a backseat in your life. Job loss is a common phenomenon at this stage as diseases associated with drinking begin developing, including liver cirrhosis and dementia. You are likely to become paranoid and fearful without any reason. Hallucinations and tremors are common side effects when attempting to stop drinking. Rehabilitation and detoxification are common avenues for helping alcoholics who are in this stage. You lose total control as the condition affects all aspects of your life including mental, social and physical life. Sleep without drinking becomes difficult. Severe cases can lead to brain damage or heart failure.

Am I an alcoholic?

It is possible to move through all the stages of alcoholism without realizing that you are becoming an alcoholic. Knowledge of who is an alcoholic is useful in identifying yourself as an alcoholic, which can be the stepping stone to seeking effective help and intervention. The definition of an alcoholic indicates that it is a person whose brain has developed a dependence on alcohol to function, whereby withdrawal symptoms manifest whenever such a person goes without a drink. Alcoholism, like most other diseases, has levels of severity.

Telling when you have crossed the line from being an average drinker to an alcoholic is not as easy as you may consider when you are the one involved. There are signs of alcoholism that may not be that obvious, and you may also tend to deny having an alcohol problem, whether consciously or subconsciously. In most cases, you will be the last person to realize an impending alcohol problem. Recognizing the symptoms of alcohol is important as this knowledge can help you fight the barrier of denial or ignorance about the problem, which can start an intervention approach. This is because the classic image of an alcoholic as a person who drinks too much and letting his life fall apart due to drinking is not always the reality. In reality, you can be a high-functioning alcoholic, but an alcoholic all the same.

Alcoholism is also regarded as alcohol use disorder due to the negative level associated with the term "alcoholism". If you have this condition, you will not be able to know when and how to stop drinking, and you can spend a great amount of time thinking about alcohol. Controlling alcohol consumption for an alcoholic is difficult, even when the condition is causing serious issues at work, home, or financially.

Signs that you may be an alcoholic

Heavy drinking is a sign of alcoholism. In men, heavy drinking involves having four or more drinks within a day. This level can be equated to more than 14 drinks within a week. heavy drinking for women is drinking over three or seven drinks within a day or week, respectively. Drinking more than the described weekly limit puts a person at risk of alcoholism.

Apart from heavy drinking, other signs act as red flags for alcoholism. These include joking about being an alcoholic to friends, family, and strangers. Not keeping up with the major responsibilities at work, school or home is another red flag for alcoholism. When you start having relationship problems related to your drinking habits and cannot quit drinking, you should worry about an alcohol problem that may be out of control. Drinking alone or during inappropriate times, such as in the morning, getting drunk unintentionally should sound an alarm.

Not remembering what you did and at which place when you were drinking is a major sign that you may be becoming an alcoholic. You may also begin having legal problems such as DUI arrests. Seeking confidence or relaxation from drinking is a common behavior among alcoholics, and so is denying drinking, hiding alcohol, and getting angry due to any confrontation about your alcohol behavior. Irritability when you have no access to alcohol or when your drinking time approaches is a major red flag. Physical manifestations such as nausea and sweating, even when not drinking are signs of an alcohol disorder.

At the Bottom of the Bottle

What can happen with an alcoholic?

When you are an alcoholic, you are always in danger of alcohol overdose, which can present various challenges to your body. An alcohol overdose occurs when your blood alcohol concentration rises to 0.008% or higher. The high alcohol content leads to a shutdown of brain areas that control basic life-supporting functions like heart rate, breathing and temperature control. Some symptoms that indicate that you are experiencing alcohol overdose include dulled responses like the lack of gag reflects, which leads to the inability to prevent choking, mental confusion, trouble breathing, clammy skin, slow heart rate, extremely low body temperature, seizure, and vomiting. In some cases, alcohol overdose leads to permanent brain damage and death. You may be able to function as normal during a blackout, but the ability to record any memories will be impaired, which means that you cannot create memories during a blackout.

The increase in blood alcohol concentration increases the risk factors that include reduced motor coordination, clouded judgment, and feeling sick. Your risk of injuries from car crashes or falls increases. You may also engage in unintended or unprotected sex, while your tendency to engage in acts of violence goes higher. A high level of blood alcohol content can lead to loss of consciousness or passing out, and amnesia or blackouts. The alcohol content can continue rising even when you are unconscious as the alcohol in the intestines and stomach enters the bloodstream. Therefore, assuming that an unconscious person can sleep off, the effect is dangerous as alcohol may continue circulating throughout the body.

Choking on your own vomit is one of the most dangerous potential impacts of alcohol overdose. In this situation, the dangerous levels of alcohol prevent the normal signals controlling automatic responses like the gag reflex, which can cause you to choke on your vomit and die from the lack of oxygen. Long-lasting brain damage can occur even when a person survives such an overdose. Regular frontal lobe damage from drinking can lead to personality and behavior impairment, as well as memory problems.

Effect on health

Alcohol affects the functioning of the brain, and in some cases, it can cause significant damage to the affected area of the brain. In this case, alcoholism affects the working of the brain and how it looks. The brain's communication pathways are the most affected so that the alcoholic's reasoning, the formation of memories, and the retention of new memories are compromised. Drinking a lot of alcohol at a time might cause paralysis, delirium, and hallucinations, as well.

Too much drinking both on a single occasion or over time causes damage to your heart and may develop into serious heart conditions such as cardiomyopathy and arrhythmias. Cardiomyopathy is the damage to the heart muscle so that it becomes stretchy and droopy, while arrhythmias is the irregular beating of the heart. The alcohol effect on the heart may also cause stroke and high blood pressure.

Alcoholism causes liver inflammation and other serious liver diseases. These diseases include: steatosis, fibrosis, alcoholic hepatitis, and cirrhosis. Your pancreas is also at risk of producing toxic substances because of alcoholism. The toxic substance produced causes serious health issues such as pancreatitis and a dangerous health condition of the blood vessels swelling in the pancreases inhibiting adequate digestion.

Research has also revealed that drinking alcohol can cause several cancers. Health report provided by the US Department of Health in the National Toxicology Program categorized alcohol as a human carcinogen. The report indicated that drinking alcohol over time increases the risk of getting alcohol-related cancers such as liver cancer, breast, esophageal, and colorectal cancer, head and neck cancer. The 2009 data released by the US department of health showed that 3.5% of deaths related to cancer are a result of alcohol. While 3.5% may seem like a small number to you, it translates to 19,500 deaths in the year 2009.

Drinking alcohol weakens your immune system increasing the likelihood of getting sick, as well as poor response to treatments. Alcoholics are more vulnerable to serious respiratory diseases such as tuberculosis and pneumonia than occasional and social drinkers. When you drink too much alcohol in one instant, your body becomes exposed to diseases for up to 24 hours after the drinking spree.

How does alcohol affect your senses?

Alcohol consumption can alter the activity in the brain leading to impacts on the functioning of the body and senses. Your brain is responsible for the proper functioning of your senses. Since alcohol can cross the blood-brain barrier, which means that it can cross from the blood circulation into the brain cells, over drinking can dull your senses as signals are not fired to the sensory cells quickly and effectively.

Alcohol has a significant fear inhibition effect. It alters your reasoning and increases your willingness to take uncalculated risks. Such an effect might result in self-injury on misjudgment in assessing safety while driving, crossing the road, or even just cooking, resulting in an accident that might cost your life.

In terms of the five common senses, alcohol affects your brain activities, causing a temporary or permanent impairment to the functioning of these senses. This is because alcohol is a depressant substance that depresses the functionality of the nerve cells in the brain. Such an effect results in delayed communication between the nerve cells and the sensory cells resulting in a slowed or ineffective response of the senses.

Sight

Blurred vision is a common symptom resulting from the consumption of large quantities of alcohol. The neurotransmitters in the brain cannot send signals for the proper functioning of the eyes, preventing you from seeing clearly. Extreme intoxications are associated with a complete lack of vision, which makes walking or driving without supervision extremely dangerous. Conditions such as temporary double vision or diplopia can be caused by overdrinking as the alcohol causes the eye muscles to lose precision, which affects your ability to focus on one object. When alcohol is consumed in a large amount, it causes blurred vision. This is because of the inability of the transmitters to send the correct signal that enables the eyes to focus. In case you are exposed to extreme levels of alcohol intoxication, you might end up losing your sight for good.

Taste and smell

A dulled sense of smell and taste occurs without our realization. The cells in the mouth and nose stop functioning at their full capacity. The excited state may make food seem to taste quite amazing, but the taste will not be nearly as good as it normally is when you are not intoxicated. Part of the reason for the loss of taste is the dryness of the tongue caused by alcohol, which is a dehydrating agent. You may also miss out on some smells as your sense of smell is impaired. The cells in the nose and mouth are affected to the extent that they fail to perform as they are required. The impaired sense of smell may pose a significant danger to the affected as they might be unable to smell leaking gas and fuel.

Touch

The sense of touch is adversely affected. The symptom of this effect is seen when you begin feeling numb in your toes and fingers. A decreased pain perception takes effect due to the dulled sense of touch due to the use of alcohol by alcoholics to reduce pain. This is a dangerous situation, as you may not notice when you have sustained an injury.

Hearing

It is possible to lose your sense of hearing after consuming large volumes of alcohol. However, this change may not be detectable when you are intoxicated, but others will notice that you laugh or talk louder than sober people. Most people have a reduced sense of hearing after drinking a large volume of alcohol.

Causes of Alcoholism

Easy access and availability

For years, regulating the availability or access to alcohol has been employed as a moderating method for alcohol problems in communities in different parts of the world. The availability of alcohol, especially for teenagers who binge drink, is enhanced by the low cost of various alcohol products hence an effort to regulate not only the access to these products but also the cost attached to them. Illicitly obtained alcohol by teenagers is associated with high levels of misuse. Alcohol obtained in controlled environments reduces the risk of binge drinking, as well as drinking in public places by teenagers. Parental provisions, which allow for parties, is also associated with easy access to alcohol by teenagers. Alcohol access can be made higher for teenagers via means such as personal purchases, as well as off-license settings proxy purchasing through adults and access through adults, parents, and family.

Alcohol availability does not affect children only as adults are also susceptible to alcoholism due to easy access. When you are developing an alcohol problem, living close to an alcohol store or a bar can increase your chances of becoming an alcoholic. Storing alcohol in the house can also increase your susceptibility to developing an alcohol problem. Parental control, including restrictions to obtaining alcohol outside parental environments, is seen as not enough in curbing teenage drinking and should be attached by providing genuine legislation, as well as enforcing activities toward reducing independence alcohol access by teenagers.

Various strategies have been used to reduce the ease of access to alcohol, including raising the minimum legal drinking age, imposing greater monopoly control efforts on alcohol sales, lowering the density of outlets, lowering the number of outlets, and limiting days and hours of sale. Lowering the minimum drinking age is associated with adverse alcohol problems, as evidenced by the case of New Zealand, where reducing the age limit from 20 to 18 in 1999 caused an increase in emergency department admissions associated with intoxication, traffic crashes and prosecutions for driving under the alcohol influence. These issues indicate that access or availability of alcohol can increase your risk of developing an alcohol disorder.

Mass media effect

The recent campaign to deglamorize alcohol is an indication of the negative impacts that glamorous alcohol advertisements through mass media have had on the promotion of alcoholism. What you are constantly exposed to through mass media can have a great influence on your behavior. The changes may be gradual at times, but long-lasting. According to research, a teenager is more susceptible to teenage drinking when exposed to television and movies depicting alcohol use. Other mass media that promote alcohol use include advertisements for various alcohol brands and music whose lyrics are about the use of alcohol. Most of the lyrics about alcohol use are also related to violence and sex. In 2009, $1.7 billion was used by the alcohol industry in media advertising, which increases penetration of messages that promote alcohol use to both youths and adults.

The fact that adolescents name alcohol brands with high advertising as their favorite brands is an indication of the influence of mass media on alcohol consumption. Alcohol advertisement has an overall effect of causing a positive attitude towards consumption, especially among teenagers. The positive portrayal of alcohol in commercials and movies is associated with stimulating people, especially the youth, to drink. It is estimated that even normal drinkers tend to consume more alcohol when exposed to movies portraying positive images about alcohol consumption. Mass media works effectively in changing your attitude about drinking.

A look into the targeted content indicates that there are gender differences in terms of the message used by alcohol brands to target users. For example, male-oriented media tend to present drinking as a means of forming friendships and masculine identity. On the other hand, mass media tends to present drinking to women in terms of celebrity and glamour, but also suggest that drinking is not as acceptable to women as it is to men. Social media is proliferated with accounts of people showing their drinking culture, which normalizes drinking and can lead you to view alcoholism as a normal or fun thing.

Boredom

Contrary to popular opinion that alcoholics are homeless people, you might be surprised to know that the growth of the well-being of people and the country is also associated with mass alcoholism. One of the consequences of well-being may be boredom as people find themselves with a lot of free time not having to work all the time to cater to their needs. Thus, some of the people who have developed an alcohol problem have been successful in the past. In the quest for more excitement, you may begin indulging in drinking, but the problem develops when you associate fun and excitement with drinking to the point where you are bored unless you are drunk. Getting bored with yourself, your life, and your job may cause you to become restless. The lack of creativity, endeavor and motivation may cause you to seek unhealthy alternatives alike alcoholism, which ultimately leads to a destructive and antisocial path of addiction. You are likely to develop an alcohol problem if your life is dull and lacking interesting or exciting activities to keep you entertained.

The Power of Our Beliefs

Why do we like to drink?

For centuries people have been drinking with reasons for that varying from one person or group to another. Most of the reasons people provide for drinking are associated with the effect of drinking on their mind and brain.

One of the reasons some people provide for drinking is that alcohol tastes nice with taste preferences varying from one individual to another. Sweet tasting alcohol may make you prone to drinking and alcohol addiction when you have a predisposition to prefer sugar. Drinking even the bitter-tasting alcoholic drinks over time leads to increasing tasty responses.

You may also drink due to a craving for alcohol caused by the release of dopamine, which controls pleasure and reward in the brain hence motivating addiction. It results in a motivation to continue drinking after your first drink, which may lead to addiction.

Drinking to feel better is one of the most common reasons people give for drinking. In this case, you use alcohol as self-medication when you want to unwind or alleviate the stress associated with the workplace or study pressure. However, acute alcohol consumption is known for stimulating stress rather than relieving it.

Alcohol acts on the prefrontal cortex, which is associated with social behavior and decision making, and you lose the self-resistance you usually have before drinking. This leads to increased sociability as your inhibitory control weakens.

Part of the reason why some people drink is that it eases pain by dulling the perception of pain. The slow neural reaction when intoxicated delays pain-causing signals from being detected by the sensory neurons. However, tolerance for alcohol as one becomes an alcoholic reduces the effect of pain relief associated with alcohol consumption.

Drinking to sleep is a common reason given by many people, as alcohol reduces the slow-wave allowing you to drop off faster. However, researchers indicate that while it may put you to sleep, the quality of sleep when intoxicated does not improve. On the contrary, the effect of alcohol on cognitive processes like memory consolidation may be detrimental to your memory processes.

Myths

The myths about the benefits of drinking alcohol are spread rapidly, with big alcohol producers taking center stage in spreading these myths. One of the long-standing myths is that a drink a day is good for your health. On the contrary, not drinking is associated with better health than drinking, even with moderation. It indicates that you can be of better health by avoiding drinking altogether.

The myth that moderate consumption of alcohol can improve the heart condition is spread all over. Alcohol consumption can increase the risk of cardiovascular disease, asthma, and allergic reactions since drinking reduces the effectiveness of your immune system.

Conditions such as dementia, asthma, obesity and diabetes increase in prevalence even through moderate drinking. Drinking alcohol can increase allergic reactions such as sneezing, a skin rash, and an itchy nose as alcohol intake tends to trigger an allergic reaction associated with the immune system.

One of the greatest myths spread by the alcohol industry to promote consumption and profits is that alcohol consumption is common, healthy, normal and responsible. This myth lead you to view drinking and over-drinking as a regular thing and the center of a healthy social life. In most cases, alcohol advertising is linked to health, sports, physical beauty, having friends, romanticism and leisure activities. On the contrary, you can have a vibrant life without depending on alcohol. Making alcohol consumption seem like a regular thing has heavily contributed to drinking beyond the recommended limit.

Another myth is that those who experience damages caused by alcohol are a small group of people who cannot handle alcohol. On the contrary, people who experience the negative effects of alcohol are ordinary people who do not have to be homeless or social deviants. This shows that regardless of your family background or socioeconomic status, the damages of alcohol can affect you. In reality, a big percentage of adult Americans do not use alcohol at all, with only the top 20% of alcohol consumers account for more than half of all alcohol consumed in a year. The message that it is abnormal not to drink is misinforming as many people leading a normal life do not drink and still afford to live a normal and interesting life.

Awareness of the problem

The secret to a full recovery from alcoholism is being aware of the problem. The kind of awareness that brings positive results is based on accepting that you have a problem and that you would like to find a solution from it. Other destructive awareness of the problem is accepting that you are neck-deep in problem, and that is it for you. As such, you must first accept that you are an alcoholic and that alcoholism is a chronic disease, not a failure on your part. From that perspective, awareness would lead to the search for a solution and the recovery process commences.

Awareness of the problem is the secret to achieving sustainable results with regards to recovery and quitting the drinking habit for good. Acceptance gives you the power to take control of your life and your decision once more. This is because you can understand your limitations and face your problems head-on.

Accept the secondary benefits as the reasons for drinking. Whether it is for improved sleep, better sex, or to fit in with your peers, it is important to know that these benefits do not measure up to the dangerous effects of alcoholism. Apart from losing control of your life, you may lose important people, destroy your career, end up with serious health issues, and in the end, lose the respect of your friends and family.

Awareness helps you to overcome the consequences of denial. These consequences range from guilt, health deuteriation, poor social and career performance, anger, shame, and self-pity. The maladaptive emotional coping is the result of the non-acceptance of alcoholism as a disease and an illness that affects you directly. Adopting a positive mindset is the first step to self-awareness and recovery.

In some cases, seeking help from professionals may result in acceptance through treatment. In the case where you decide that you are no longer capable of helping yourself and seeking professional help in the form of support groups or rehabilitative services, you gain awareness of the issue and the extent to which it has an affect you.

While taking some professionally prescribed medicines can help you to stop or reduce drinking, motivational enhancement, and cognitive-behavioral therapies are also useful in enhancing your sobriety success and preventing relapse.

Note that you can only get help when you have some level of awareness that you have a problem. The significance of awareness is apparent because acceptance doesn't mean that you like your situation, but rather admitting your limitations and resolving to do the necessary to overcome an illness that is destroying your life.

Reasons to Quit Drinking

Drinking may seem fun until the negative consequences take hold of your life. The supposed benefits of drinking cannot compare with the benefits you get when you quit drinking. As much as quitting can seem impossible, especially when you are an alcohol addict, the staggering number of people who have successfully quit drinking is enough evidence that quitting is not that far-fetched. Quitting takes only a few steps, but the benefits are amazing. Here are a few benefits of why you should quit drinking.

Feeling better

The great misconception about drinking is that alcohol makes you feel better. Binge and chronic drinking are quite dangerous, and you will realize that you will feel much better when you stop drinking. The feeling is attributed to the ability of alcohol to numb the brain so that when you stop drinking, your neurotransmitters normalize, and neuron communication stabilizes as your body saves on energy used to process alcohol.

Excessive drinking causes your liver to go into overdrive mode to metabolize the alcohol while your brain also works overtime to calibrate the effects. Irregular speeds of pumping are recorded in the heart and lungs, which is far from how the body was designed to work. These side effects can be eliminated when you stop drinking as the body is free from processing these toxic chemicals, which allow you to focus your energy on more productive things as your body functions optimally.

Quitting prevents you from making regrettable decisions such as unintentional sex when you are intoxicated. The shame and guilt accompanied by drinking become a thing of the past. You could expect to start feeling better within a short time after you have quit drinking, especially is this action is accompanied by healthy eating and exercising.

Looking younger

One of the negative attributes of alcohol is that it is a diuretic, which means that it has the ability to dehydrate the skin, which reduces skin elasticity. When you quit drinking, the collagen levels of your skin are restored slowly while redness disappears. The dehydration affects you by making you look older as your skin dried out, becoming less elastic. Collagen is an important protein connecting your skin cells while also strengthening the tissues. The breakdown of collagen by alcohol makes your skin look saggy and loose.

Body tissue inflammation is another effect associated with drinking, which is responsible for getting flushed in the face while drinking for some people. Inflation of the skin causes these flashes, which can damage your skin over time due to constant inflammation.

According to researches, excessive drinking causes aging of body cells, which reduces the lifespan of cells in the liver, skin, heart, and other organs. The aging of your body prevents it from producing new cells as your skin ages, and most of your organs begin deteriorating faster. You can get your healthiest skin and look better when you quit drinking.

Saving money

An average of 4.5 million Americans purchased alcohol worth $200 every week, which indicates that alcohol cessation has benefits that supersede physical gains and include financial benefits like saving money. A few bottles of wine or beer may not be costly, but the cost of alcohol adds up when you drink daily or weekly. In addition, you tend to become irrational in financial decisions when drunk. A large amount of money you spend on alcohol, when compounded, can go into beneficial uses.

Social stability

Heavy drinking is associated with high peer-nominated status. In reality, many people are socially isolated due to their drinking problems and people end up feeling alone, ashamed, and guilty. The booze can make you forget that there are people in the world who would treat you with love and connect with you. The lack of connection is usually associated with alcohol addiction as alcohol gives an addict a sense of stability.

When you are an avoidant individual, you indulge more in alcohol consumption to avoid painful emotions, as well as self-awareness. However, these connections formed by drinking are not real as a real personal human connection can only be developed through sobriety forcing you to develop real human connections.

Losing weight

Second only to fat itself, which has a calorie content of 9 per gram, alcohol has almost double the calorie level of most carbohydrates and proteins at a calorie level of 7 per gram. Quitting drinking can be one of the best strategies for losing weight. Alcohol is processed as sugar by the body before being converted to fat, giving drinkers more weight compared to non-drinkers. A close relationship between obesity and excessive consumption of alcohol has also been established.

Losing weight is associated with several benefits. Other than the calories gained from alcohol itself, drinking gives you a craving for high-carb foods, which act as a cure for a hangover. The high-carb food results in more weight gain, which can reach a dangerous level.

A healthy heart

Approximately 510,000 people in the US die every year because of heart disease, which accounts for a quarter of all deaths. You can lower the danger of heart attack by recovering from alcoholism. Habitual drinking tends to increase the danger of experiencing heart disease, especially if you are prone to pulmonary conditions. A healthier heart is possibly the greatest benefit you get by quitting alcohol. Alcohol increases the risk of a heart disease by increasing the fat level in your bloodstream through an increased level of cholesterol. These levels reduce the speed of blood circulation through your body, making the heart work harder to pump blood. Heart failure is the result of high cholesterol levels over time.

Gain time for taking up new activities

Since drinking requires time allocation both during drinking and recovering. You will discover that you have a lot of time when you quit drinking. This time can be used to take up new productive and fun activities. You may have several hours to take an extra shift for additional income, or simply relax and watch a movie.

After quitting, most people realize they had hobbies that they did not know about. Quitting gives you a quest state of mind to live in the moment, self-rediscover yourself, and engage in any activity that you are interested in. Finding a new hobby is important in sustaining sobriety. While exercises and book reading are some of the activities you can take up, there is no limit to what you can do. The trick is to evade staying home idle and alone on Saturday or Friday nights or so to speak.

While focusing is a challenge among heavy drinkers and alcohol, quitting will increase your attention and focus on tasks and other activities, making it easier for you to enjoy simple activities such as cooking and baking. You will also enjoy spending time with your family and people that you respect. This is because alcoholism has a way of making you avoid your family and close friends who do not drink because of feeling criticized, judge, or simply unappreciated. Alcoholism makes it easy to disappoint people who had hope in you and those that you strive to make them proud. For this reason, it is easy for you to avoid them rather than see them at all costs. Guess what, quitting removes this burden and allows you to interact with anybody that you would like to in a respectful and fun way.

Being sober gives you a chance to right all the wrongs of the past. Since alcohol makes people prone to offending others and making mistakes, quitting drinks gives you a fresh start. Quitting is the ultimate tangible proof that you regret the wrongs done in the past, making people more willing to give you a second chance.

Health improvement

In the year 2014, 1900 deaths were caused by liver diseases caused by alcohol in the US alone. Quitting drinking will save you loads of health problems. The liver issue is the first in the list because the body is not meant to process alcohol, hence consumption of alcohol makes the liver work the extra mile to process it, causing cirrhosis and hepatitis. Luckily enough, the liver can regenerate itself. When you stop drinking, the liver generates new cells to correct any damages incurred during the drinking period.

While some people take alcohol because it improves their sleep, researches indicate that alcoholics who started to drink so they can sleep better, end up suffering from insomnia when they abuse alcohol and become an alcoholic. The good news is that this harmful effect of alcohol can be reversed when you stop drinking.

The delta activity in the brain triggered by alcohol is useful in memory restoration and learning, however, it also triggers the alpha activities that take place when people are awake. These two effects counteract to cause insomnia or reduced quality of sleep. Insomnia and low quality of sleep cause fatigue, poor concentration, and low ability to focus, absent-mindedness, and some mental health issues such as depression. When you stop drinking, you will get your sleep back sooner or later, depending on the duration in which you had insomnia.

Focus on personal achievements and development

Alcoholism comes with many issues that make it difficult for you to concentrate on your personal goals. Between all the illnesses, hangovers, and fatigue, you can hardly find time to regroup and plan for your development and self-improvement.

Quitting improves your sense of wellbeing and your quality of life. This is because it improves your emotional, economic, and physical health, giving you optimal conditions to be productive, to engage in positive social interaction, and to adopt healthy lifestyle choices.

Why Quitting Can Be So Hard?

There is no magic pill

There is a tendency among alcoholics who want to recover from the disorder to seek the easy way out. Unfortunately, there is no magic pill that could make the problem vanish away as you have to go through the process of overcoming alcohol addiction the right way. This tendency to seek an easy way out has led to many users relapsing repeatedly. Since alcohol addiction takes a long time to develop, healing takes equally long with the risk of relapse in forcing the addict to work hard in maintaining sobriety. Below are some of the primary reasons why quitting can be so hard.

Admitting you have a problem

One of the hardest parts of facing your alcohol problem is admitting that you have a problem. In most cases, you are the last person to acknowledge that you have a serious alcohol addiction. You may admit that you like to have a drink, but admitting your need to drink can be hard. A common observation is the tendency to tell people who are close to you that you can stop drinking whenever you want.

Also, you may be aware of your drinking problem, but you become scared of quitting. This fear may have been provoked by efforts to stop drinking before, which you found quite tough with loved ones telling you just to stop thinking that it is easy on you. It is prudent to point out that there would be no addicts if stopping was that easy. Most people who have no experience with addiction think that the problem can be ended by simply quitting. However, this notion is further from the truth, especially for those who have experienced addiction.

It is easier for an addict to deny having an alcohol problem than to try quitting. Another strategy used widely is blaming other people for your drinking problem or finding excuses as to why you are unable to quit at the moment. You will soon realize that your health and relationships are reaching a damaging point by continuing to drink.

Fear of recovery

Getting help for alcoholism can be a scary thing due to the fear of rehabilitation. The stories of unpleasant withdrawal symptoms further activate the fear for rehabilitation compounded by your previous efforts to quit, which were futile.

It is important that you realize that quitting alcohol is tough but possible. Your body's dependence on alcohol means that you will crave it when you try quitting. However, many excellent treatment centers exist all over the country, which offer safe detoxification. Medical supervision is conducted efficiently at these centers with appropriate medication given for dealing with the symptoms. The fear of new and unknown can be overwhelming, but the possibility of living a free life from addiction should be more compelling.

Brain changes

The difficulty of quitting drinking is related to the intensity and length of substance use. The longer you have been drinking, the harder it becomes to quit mainly due to changes in your brain. Three major changes occurred in the brain that makes it so hard to quit as dependency develops. During the initial stages of drinking, alcohol stimulates dopamine release, which is associated with rewarding and pleasurable activities such as having sex and enjoying a good meal. Dopamine stimulates your interest in enjoying alcohol, and you end up drinking more to the point where your brain associated alcohol with these positive experiences.

A second change occurs in your brain as you continue drinking. Your brain's sensitivity to dopamine release increases over time, causing fading of alcohol; enjoyment. Alcohol tolerance means that you will need to drink more to feel good. The transition for drinking to alcohol addiction occurs at this point.

In the third stage, your brain's repeated exposure to alcohol leads to changes to compensate for the depressant nature of alcohol. The slowing effect of alcohol activates the release of an excitatory chemical called glutamate in the brain to counter the slowing effect of alcohol. More excitement develops in the brain, which remains in the excited state even when you are not drinking. This excited state is associated with anxiety, problems sleeping, and tremors. You continue drinking to obtain the depressant effect of alcohol to counter the excited state, and the cycle of drinking continues.

These changes in the brain may become permanent if you have been drinking for years. Neurological changes take place in the brain with chronic use of alcohol as certain brain circuits become sensitized, which leads to changes in neurotransmitter levels. The changes can affect the executive function of the brain, which affects the decision-making aspect that you normally use to stop drinking. At this point, it means that you may need to avoid alcohol use for the rest of your life.

Family history and genetics accounts for approximately half of alcohol use disorder cases. The other half of these cases are attributed to environmental exposure with environmental factors such as social influences by family and friends, age when you had your first drink, and access and availability of alcohol contributing to the cases of this disorder.

If you are someone with a long-term addiction problem, quitting can be a complicated process, and you may have a high chance of relapse. However, you must be hopeful due to the treatable nature of chronic alcoholism through a combination of counseling and medication.

Rules to Follow on This Path

The danger of relapse when you start your journey to recovery is high. However, recovery is possible by following a few basic rules, which are easy to remember. These are the rules you should observe.

First rule: change your lifestyle

You cannot achieve recovery by simply not using alcohol. You need to create a new lifestyle where consumption of alcohol is not easy. Changing your life is important since it prevents factors contributing to your addiction from catching up with you.

Hoping that you will not have to change your life on your path to recovery is futile. When you try to recover while maintaining your old lifestyle, your chances of relapse increase. Developing a positive mindset for recovery by viewing it as an opportunity for change can be more powerful as opposed to viewing the need for change as something negative. Necessary changes can improve the quality of your life and increase your happiness and well-being. The silver lining that comes with addiction is that recovery forces you to evaluate your life and make changes, which you may not have considered when you were a non-addict.

The idea of change can be overwhelming when you are trying to recover. However, change does not have to be everything in your life as only a small part of your life will need to be changed. Three categories of change are necessary. The first category is changing your negative thinking patterns. The second category involves avoiding things, places, and people you associate with alcoholism. The third category is a conscious decision to incorporate the rules of recovery.

Second rule: be completely honest

Lying is necessary for addiction as you begin lying about getting your alcohol, hiding it, and planning your next relapse. You are also prone to deny the consequences of alcoholism as you begin lying to yourself. Emotional relapse occurs when you feel you are incapable of becoming completely honest. One of the challenges you should overcome on your path to recovery is telling the truth and admitting when the truth is misspoken while making the necessary corrections.

It can be quite challenging to define the level of honesty in a group that does not jeopardize your work relationships. Consider that the path to recovery involves a group comprising of doctors, family, counselors, sponsors, and self-help groups. Telling the truth can be hard, but complete honesty is required for a full recovery. You can expand your circle as you become more honest with yourself and others. Honesty is preferred at all times except when it harms others.

Third rule: ask for help

At first, you may try quitting addiction on your own while attempting to prove to yourself and others that you are in control of your addiction. However, you can increase your chance of long-term recovery by joining a self-help group. Combining a self-help group and substance abuse program can be more effective in recovery.

Groups such as Alcoholics Anonymous (AA) and Adult Children of Alcohol (ACA) are spread across the country in almost every town. Regular meeting attendance is the best way for getting maximum help from these groups. Participating in such groups provides many benefits such as eliminating the feeling of loneliness, hearing the voice of addiction from others, and learning from others about recovery. These groups offer a safe place of no judgment, which removes the fear of guilt and shame that acts as an obstacle to recovery.

Fourth rule: practice self-care

Understanding the importance of self-care begins with an understanding of why you use alcohol with some of the common reasons for using alcohol, including to reward yourself, relax or escape. Understanding these reasons can help you in finding alternatives since it is easy to overlook self-care on your path to recovery. Without self-care initiatives, going to self-help groups may not be effective in preventing relapse. The difficulty of self-care is attributed to the tendency to be too self-critical as a recovering addict.

The difference between self-care and selfishness is that selfishness entails taking more than you need while self-care entails taking as much as you need. Taking less help than you need can result in exhausting and relapse to escape or relax. You should realize that being good to others begins with being good to yourself.

Fifth rule: do not bend the rules

This rule reminds you to stop resisting and sabotaging change by insisting on recovering your way. Looking for loopholes in recovery is the first test that you are bending the rules. Asking for professional help and ignoring the advice given should be a warning sign that you are bending the rules.

The goal is to acknowledge the fun you derived from using, become eager to begin a new chapter in your life free for alcohol addiction.

The Ups and Downs of Real People

While building your personal motivation for quitting drinking, it will be useful to know that you are not alone on the path. Below some real stories from AA are provided, the ups and downs of real people, the difficulties they faced on the way of overcoming alcohol addiction. The names are hidden for confidentiality purposes.

It is never too late

The hero of the story is a metallurgist, he is 36 years old, was married for 2 years. His alcohol experience is comparable to his work experience, comprises 19 years. The man tasted alcohol for the first time when he was 3 years old, when parents gave him a sip of liquor at the festive table. He remembers that he was drunk for the first time while celebrating the first college day with his friends. The next morning, future metallurgist's head was literally cracking and then someone suggested to have some hair of the dog to feel fresh again. And from that moment it all started. Almost every evening ended up with a drinking party and several times with fights. The metallurgist even had to spend some time in a drug clinic. Nevertheless, neither the cries of the relatives, nor the advice of friends, nor even the threats of the bosses helped, and alcohol was becoming more and more solid in the life of this person. That was until doctors diagnosed the liver cirrhosis. It sounds scary, but thanks to liver disease, the man managed to hold out without alcohol for 3 months. And it seemed that life began to get better, passions at work calmed down, his daily activity returned to its usual rhythm. Everything seemed to take its course, but one day the metallurgist felt that he sorely lacked adrenaline. The consequences of the first glass after a long break were terrible, after a fight in the dark corner, the man miraculously survived. His whole life could have fallen into the abyss, but it did not, thanks to his childhood friend, who accidentally returned to the city. That friend literally forced the man to visit the narcologist, and then join the AA. It is incredible, but only the support of the friend along with the stories of other people helped to gain faith in the life of this person. There is nothing shameful in the profession of a metallurgist, but the hero of this story is now obtaining a degree in law. Learning as well as getting on the feet is never too late!

Fight for your family

Our second hero is engineer, he is 28 years old, alcoholic for 5 years. An incredibly talented guy who loves his job and, even more, loves to drink. Initially, the CEO of the company, in which he worked, believed that specifically this person can even be allowed to drink at the workplace, he was so indispensable, had truly golden hands. The engineer willingly used this "benefit" until he got drunk to the point of delirium tremens right at the workplace. He was immediately fired of course. Alcoholism started at his student years. He was dating several girls. Our hero kicked out the first ones because he believed that they were "sawing" him. The latter girl stayed with him for a long time exactly because she did not saw, but could sometimes drink with him and keep him a company. The engineer still lives with that girl and believes that she is the one who helped him to change the perception of the world. The thing is that the girl could have a few drinks with him, but at the same time, she could easily not drink at all just because she did not want to. This really hurt his pride: "A girl may not drink if she does not want to, while I am a man living in the power of a glass." The engineer tried to quit drinking, but every time relapsed terribly. He had 3 epileptic fits, and the last one was critical, the man began to suffocate. His girlfriend managed to call the ambulance just in time, and that way saved his life. The engineer has not been drinking for a year, and he is going to marry that girl.

There is no shame in seeking help

Student, 21 years old, alcoholic for 3 years, single. Reckless youth forced the guy to try not only alcohol but also amphetamines. Though the consumption of the last was short because once when he was on drugs, he barely bashed in the skull of his best friend. Alcohol easily replaced drugs. At one of the housewarming parties, the student got drunk till almost losing his pulse. On the way home, he vomited right in the taxi, and the night was very hard for him. The guy understood that it was pointless and disgusting to continue pursuing such a lifestyle. Actually, it was hard to continue since every time after drinking, he ended up in a narcological clinic. Serious problems with the university were added to this. As a result, that housewarming party became the last point of alcohol consumption in his life. The painful process of struggling with himself began. For a while, it seemed for the student that his life had lost all its meaning. He could not imagine joy without a beer or wine. Nothing was satisfying. But our guy was lucky and managed to meet a practicing narcologist, who forced him to drink 3 capsules with a pep talk: "If you are planning to drink at least a drop of alcohol in the next 6 months, you would better create a testament right now". These words had a striking effect on the student. He has not been drinking for 5 months and will soon visit that narcologist again. Fortunately, he saved the business card.

Find your passion

Saleswoman, 34 years old, divorced and has a daughter. She has been drinking for 8 years every week, but strongly disagreed with the "alcoholic" label, despite the fact that she had to pawn family jewels several times and occasionally was admitted to the hospital. Woman grows up a daughter, for whom the mother's example is disgusting from a young age. The woman drunk several times till delirium tremens, and she beat her daughter like crazy. As a result, the grandmother and grandfather took the girl to protect her. Things changed for the worse. The woman came to the psychiatric clinic, where she was diagnosed with schizophrenia. After some time, the voices in her head stopped, and she was finally discharged. She started to understand that she could not cope with her problems on her own. She decided to seek entertainment on the world wide web and wanted to chat with someone on dating sites. But accidentally she found a travelers' club. One of the rules of this club was: no alcohol. Her first outing was a small hike. And, you guessed it, she quit drinking. In the near future, the woman is going to fly to Tibet and then to Cuba with her daughter.

Make changes happen in 5 steps

Build motivation

Half of your success to recovery will be determined by the goals you set for yourself. Setting drinking limits to no more than 2 standard drinks if you are a healthy male adult below the age of 65 and no more than one drink, if you are a healthy adult woman or a man older than 65 per day, are below the recommended guidelines. You can set your drinking goals with your doctor in the event that these limits are too high due to your age or certain medical conditions.

Your goals can also include other concrete personal motivations, such as the need to prolong your life and the joy of being conscious every time. Putting these goals in writing by listing the reasons you want to quit alcohol, including to sleep better, improve your relationships, or feeling healthier, can act as a powerful motivation whenever you take a look at these written goals. Keeping a diary of your drinking can also be a powerful motivation to stop. Ideally, you can keep a diary during the first four weeks of your recovery to track information about how much your drink, what you drink, and where. Comparing this information with your goal can alert you about the troubles you are having with sticking to your goals, which you can then discuss with their doctor or any other health professionals. Goal setting with a positive mindset is a vital part of recovery that will set off your recovery process or success.

Avoid temptation

One of the weaknesses in your recovery path will be constant temptations to relapse. Therefore, steering clear of places and people that draw you to drinking should be one of the first changes you make. You should develop a plan in advance to help you manage how to deal with events you associate with drinking, such as vacations and holidays. Monitoring your feelings should also become part of your strategy since feelings of loneliness, worry and anger can tempt you to grab a drink. Cultivating new ways of coping with stress, such as establishing a new circle of friends, can be useful in warding off temptation.

The temptation to relapse can be caused by high-risk conditions such as anger, hunger, tiredness, and loneliness. Most of these high-risk circumstances occur at the end of the day as you become hungry for not eating, lonely due to isolation, angry for having a tough day, and tired because of the day's events. The high-risk situations can also include different types of people likely drinking buddies and people with whom you are in conflict. Places from which you drink or buy alcohol should also be avoided. You should also avoid things reminding you of alcohol.

Awareness of these high-risk situations will help you steer clear to avoid being caught off-guard. You can also engage in better self-care, including eating healthier, joining a support group where you do not feel isolated, developing better sleep habits to avoid getting tired, and learning to relax to avoid feelings of resentment and anger.

Practice self-consciousness

When you finally decide to quit drinking, it is of ultimate importance for you to be aware of your needs and priorities at all times. You will have to make a conscious decision to stand against the pressure so that you do not drink because of the company or anybody's expectations. In this case, you will have to inform your family and close friends about your decision to quit drinking. By sharing with friends and close family members about your intention to quit drinking, they will understand the reasons why you constantly turn down the drinking offers and other invitations to go partying. They will be motivated to help you overcome the urge to relapse.

Since quitting might be a gradual process, it is advisable that you only drink when you have made a conscious decision about it and not influenced in any way by circumstances. Gradually reducing your alcohol intake is associated with numerous health benefits as it prevents the development of the withdrawal syndrome. Unfortunately, for most alcoholics, there is no stopping once you have started drinking. At this point, it is advisable to give up alcohol completely. Nonetheless, the use of alcohol-free days works for most heavy drinking. For example, if you went drinking every day, you could start by drinking on a three-day per week basis, then change it to weekends only, and in the end, you will be able to pull off from the drinking habit altogether.

Pursue the self-development goal

Your decision to stop drinking and recover from alcoholism is an indication of your intention to become a better person. Setting self-development goals is a key in quitting. These developmental goals will be a point of focus and motivation for you. You can take up exercise to lose extra weight. By so doing, time and effort spent in working out and tracking your progress will motivate you to keep improving your health and wellbeing.

It is also advisable to make other financial goals, such as buying a house or a car. The savings and extra working hours put in achieving this goal will not only result in getting the coveted house but also instill discipline, work ethic, and focus on the important things in life.

You could also decide to improve your relationship with your children and other family members. Spending time with the people you love motivates you to become a better person in every aspect of your living.

Another way that self-development can be implemented in your life is through the reward system. Whenever you achieve a quitting target such as the consistent reduction of drinking-days and the amount of alcohol consumed in those days, you could reward yourself. The rewards should be progressive based on the milestones achieved by getting one of the things that make you happy, such as a weekend getaway to some relaxing and fancy destinations, or that dress or watches that you have been eyeing for a while.

Willpower only does not work

For you to get fully recovered, you must have a strong support system to help you out when you are not able to work things out by yourself. This is because following all provided steps and ensuring that you make stackable progress can be exhausting and emotionally draining experience sometimes.

While willpower is a significant part of your recovery progress, it cannot work in exclusion. Willpower will give you the motivation to make the big leaps and stay motivated, but it will not help you when you are feeling low and drained by fatigue and a strong urge to take just a sip of the drink again.

The alcoholics' support group is an effective support system because you get to relate with other people facing the same problem as you also get a sponsor to mentor you directly into sobriety. There is nothing more motivating, like knowing the challenges and victories of the people who are facing the challenge that you are facing.

The healthcare facility can also offer you a strong support system by providing professional care and medication that helps you to cope and recover from alcoholism. However, your best support system is your friends and family. Having family and friends who understand your struggle and are willing to help you get through is very motivating and effective in gaining sustainable progress towards full recovery.

Conclusion

Alcohol addiction is a disease like any other. This means that you should not be ashamed of admitting your addiction as the first process towards recovery. However, like most other diseases, alcohol addiction is treatable through a combination of therapy and medication. The road to recovery from alcohol addiction is long and complicated. Complete recovery entails measures such as creating a new life where you eliminate components of your old life that drove you to alcohol addiction. Without making a conscious decision to change these elements of your life, you will have increased your chances of relapse since these components can draw you back to drinking. The process of relapse is gradual and can begin weeks or even months before you actually pick up your first drink. Before the physical stage of relapse comes the emotional and mental phases, with the common denominator being poor self-care. Treatment of an alcohol addiction problem aims at helping you to recognize early warning signs that you are about to relapse, which will help with developing coping skills to prevent the relapse process. With treatment, your chances of recovery are increased, especially when you adhere to the five basic rules of recovery, discussed in this book.

Your addiction gives you the chance to change your life for the better. In many cases, addicts who are committed to recovery end up developing a healthier life than their life before addiction. This aspect of recovery makes it even more rewarding and prevents you from sleepwalking through your life, wondering why you are unhappy. Using this opportunity for change will enable you to look back at your life after recovery when you realize that it was the best decision you made in life. In the end, the internal peace and tranquility you will achieve after recovery may make you want to feel grateful for having an addiction in the first place. The process is slow, but the good news is that relapse is rare after five years of abstinence. Make a conscious decision to quit drinking and begin your journey toward freedom today. I totally believe in you!

www.ingramcontent.com/pod-product-compliance
Lightning Source LLC
Chambersburg PA
CBHW070335240526
45466CB00027B/1993